THE HOLLYWOOD EMERGENCY DIET

THE HOLLYWOOD EMERGENCY DIET

By
Frank Downing
with Oleg Bardoff

Copyright 1978 Millburn Book Corp.

THE HOLLYWOOD EMERGENCY DIET

TABLE OF CONTENTS

	Introduction	
	Chapter I	My Day of Reckoning
The Bad News	Chapter II	The Secret Truth About Fat People
	Chapter III	Metabolism - When it Goes Down Our Weight Goes Up
	Chapter IV	The Worst Addiction in the World
The Good News	Chapter V	The Miracle of Fructose
	Chapter VI	Turning Up the Furnace
	Chapter VII	Breaking Up the Cycle of Suffering
	Chapter VIII	Some Additional Weapons
	Chapter IX	Summary and Plan of Attack
	Chapter X	Diet Days
	Chapter XI	Eating Days
	Chapter XII	Putting it Together Step-By-Step
	Chapter XIII	The Greatest Beauty Secret in the World
	Chapter XIV	Hints from Hollywood
	Chapter XV	Getting Into Your New Role

WARNING!!!

The diet plans explained in this book have been carefully researched and they have been used by thousands of people without ill effects.

However, *every* diet plan and *every* food is dangerous for somebody.

Even staples such as milk, potatoes, orange juice and bread are contraindicated for certain people.

The information presented here is based upon the latest up-to-date scientific, diet, health, and nutritional information available. Even though the information presented here is based upon natural food substances, the author or publisher assumes no liability resulting from its application.

Always consult a doctor where matters of health are concerned.

This diet is no exception. It is especially important that you get your doctor's assurance that the fructose will not aggravate any blood sugar abnormalities you may have such as hypoglycemia or diabetes.

Even though fructose does not produce an insulin response as does sugar and is much healthier for you than sugar, if you suffer from hypoglycemia or diabetes you may not be able to use fructose or any sugar substance as outlined in this diet.

INTRODUCTION

One day last summer (1977) I went to the track at Hollywood High School for my daily 6 mile run.

As I was slowly going around the track, I noticed a guy I hadn't seen there before. He was going even slower than I was and he could only go a few yards until he had to stop and rest.

The reason was obvious. He was hideously overweight. He had an enormous gut and every time I passed him I could hear him gasping for breath.

I didn't really pay much attention to him. All I can remember is feeling sorry for the poor guy and thinking that he looked ridiculous in his running outfit.

The next day he showed up again and in the days that followed, he kept coming. After awhile I began to notice that every time I went to the track, he was there also.

He wasn't much of an athlete but he sure had determination.

One day just for the hell of it I struck up a conversation with him. He told me he was desperately trying to lose weight because his doctors had told him he was on the verge of having a heart attack. Not only that, he said he had recently gotten divorced and he was ashamed of the way he looked.

My heart went out to him.

At that time I was doing some research on weight loss systems and I told him about some new diet ideas I had discovered. He listened carefully and decided to give those ideas a try.

The results were amazing.

So far he has lost more than 55 pounds and now he can jog for an hour without stopping. His blood pressure has dropped from a dangerous 160/120 to a perfect 120/80. He has a whole new outlook on life and, to say the least, his doctors are pleased.

I am happy for him.

When I first met Frank Downing he was a fat, friendly, middle-aged actor with a lot of hope and a lot of heart.

Now he is a *thin,* friendly, middle-aged actor with a lot of hope and a lot of heart.

This book then is the story of one courageous man who has turned his life around and the remarkable diet that has helped him do it.

A Friend

CHAPTER I

MY DAY OF RECKONING

I knew I was fat.

The scales said so. The mirror said so. My doctor said so. I also knew it was bad to be fat. Bad for my career. Bad for my love life. Bad for my health.

But somehow I was able to ignore all this.

But one day, something happened that I just could not ignore. I was sitting in a screening room at MGM waiting to see the daily rushes of my electrocution scene in "Coma." Suddenly, there I was, up on that screen, ten times larger than life with my gut hanging over my belt and every detail of my immense bloated body exposed by a camera that didn't have the mercy to lie.

I was ashamed.

However, that moment has turned out to be a major turning point of my life. That image up on that screen was simply too large to ignore. It really woke me up.

I made up my mind right then and there that come hell or high water I was going to lose every ounce of my ugly fat. I wanted back my self-respect. I didn't know how I was going to do it but I knew that somehow I *was* going to do it.

The very next day I got myself a running outfit and went to Hollywood High School and started stumbling around the track.

After a couple of weeks, a man who ran at the track regularly, struck up a conversation with me. When I told him I was trying to lose weight, he told me about some amazing weight loss methods that were being used successfully by other people in Hollywood.

I began to investigate some of the things that he told me about. That was the start of my education.

The rest of this book is about the Hollywood weight loss secrets that I have learned and how they have transformed my life. And how hopefully, if you are overweight, they may also transform yours.

The next three chapters are about what I believe to be the three main stumbling blocks for anyone who is trying to lose weight. This is the bad news.

However, don't despair. The rest of the book contains the good news about how to overcome these three major problems. And in addition, some health and beauty secrets that I'll bet you have never heard about.

Hollywood, as you know, has some of the healthiest and best looking people on the face of this earth. They have to be that way. Their jobs depend on it.

As soon as you turn the page you will start to learn some of our secrets.

CHAPTER II

THE SECRET TRUTH ABOUT FAT PEOPLE

Fat people are not like skinny people.

They feel differently, they think differently, and most importantly, in most cases, their body chemistry is different!

Quite often, it is this body chemistry difference that makes a fat person fat and *keeps* him fat.

However, if you understand this important difference and how to handle it, you will find that losing weight can be a lot easier than you ever dreamed possible.

Here is an example of this difference at work.

Let's say that you and one of your naturally skinny friends want to take in a movie. Both of you are in the mood for a good thriller. So after checking the papers you decide to see "Coma."

About half way through the movie, both of you start to get hungry. Right after the part where the fat maintenance man gets brutally electrocuted, you both begin to feel really uncomfortable so one of you goes to the snack bar and comes back with a couple of big candy bars.

After you eat the candy, neither of you is hungry any more and now you can give your full attention to the movie.

However, by the time the movie has reached its exciting surprise ending, something strange has happened.

Your friend is still satisfied but you are hungry all over again—even more so than you were before.

How can this be? What's going on here? Why is it

that you are hungry while at the same time and under the same circumstances your lucky friend remains comfortably satisfied?

To solve this little mystery the first thing you need to know is why you got hungry in the first place.

It is really quite simple. You get hungry when your blood sugar is low. It's not so much how empty your stomach is that makes you hungry. It's how empty your bloodstream is of sugar. When your blood sugar drops below a certain level, your body starts sending out hunger signals. These hunger signals will cause you to be uncomfortable until you get that blood sugar level back up where it belongs.

It is very easy to raise your blood sugar level. All you have to do is eat. And the fastest way, of course, is to eat something that contains sugar. Those candy bars were just perfect for the job. They contained more than enough sugar to zoom your blood sugar level right back up to normal. In fact, they contained so much sugar that your blood sugar level rose *above* normal.

Now the trouble begins.

You see, all that extra sugar in your bloodstream causes your body to produce insulin. Insulin is used to regulate the level of sugar in your blood. If your blood sugar level gets *too* high, the insulin will remove the *extra* sugar in your bloodstream and store it in your liver for later use.

At least that's the way it is supposed to work. And it does. At least it does for people like your friend who have more or less normal body chemistry.

But unfortunately, for many fat people, it just doesn't work that way. When a fat person's blood sugar gets too high, his body has a tendency to produce *too much insulin too fast!*

This causes not only the *extra* sugar but in some cases nearly *all* of the sugar to be removed from the blood.

Guess what happens then?

You are right. Since nearly *all* the sugar is pulled out of the fat person's bloodstream, *he becomes hungry all over again!*

And what does he have to do to get his blood sugar back up to where he is no longer hungry?

Right again, He's gotta eat.

And then, of course, it starts all over again—a vicious cycle that keeps the poor fat person hungry almost all of the time.

That's why you were hungry when the movie was over and your friend was not.

His body only produced enough insulin to pull the *extra* sugar out of his bloodstream. When he walked out of the movie, his blood sugar level was normal.

On the other hand, *your* body produced so much insulin that when *you* walked out of the movie, your blood sugar wasn't normal at all—it was, in fact, considerably below normal.

And that, in a nutshell, is why you walked out hungry and he walked out happy.

Now you know the secret truth about fat people.

THEY ARE HUNGRY!

They are hungry almost all the time and it is not their fault. They are often simply the unlucky victims of a screwed-up body chemistry.

But we can change this around. Now we have a new weapon to fight this problem. You will learn all about this later on in the "Good News" section of this book. But right now please go on to Chapter III where you will learn about another little known problem shared by many people who are overweight.

CHAPTER III

METABOLISM - WHEN IT GOES DOWN OUR WEIGHT GOES UP

Let's see if you can guess the answer to the following question.

Suppose you are 25 years old and you weigh 150 pounds. You jog 20 miles each week and your food intake averages 2,800 calories, how much will you weigh 10 years from now if you stick to this exact routine?

In other words, how much will you weigh on your 35th birthday if everything stays the same?

Will you still weigh 150 pounds? A little more? A little less?

The answer may surprise you.

Under the above conditions, by the time you are 35 you will weigh more than 310 pounds!

Here's why:

Every human being has a certain amount of natural vital energy that is used to accomplish various important tasks. This is the life-force that keeps us going.

Part of this energy is used to regulate our temperature. Part of it is used for such things as the healing of cuts and wounds and the knitting back together of broken bones.

That part of this life-force that is used to turn food into energy is referred to as our metabolism.

On the average, our metabolism decreases about 1% a year every year after we reach the age of 25.

If we do not eat 1% less each year after we turn 25, then our metabolism won't be high enough to turn all that we eat into energy. And, of course, that part of our food intake that we are unable to burn as energy will be stored inside our bodies as fat deposits.

What this means is that at age 26 you must eat 1% less than you did at age 25 if you want your weight to stay the same. At 35 you must eat 10% less. At 50 you must eat 25% less. And so on.

You can see how this adds up if you will take a moment to study the figures below. (Please bear in mind that each pound of fat contains 3,500 calories.)

A	B	C	D
Age	Daily Caloric Intake	% of Calories Stored as Fat Each Day	Number of Calories Stored as Fat Each Day
25	2800	0%	0
26	2800	1%	28
27	2800	2%	56
28	2800	3%	84
29	2800	4%	112
30	2800	5%	140
31	2800	6%	168
32	2800	7%	196
33	2800	8%	224
34	2800	9%	252
35	2800	10%	280

E	F	G	H
Number of Calories Stored as Fat this Year (D x 365)	Number of pounds gained This Year (E - 3500)	Total Weight Gain so far (since age 25)	Weight at End of Year
0	0	0	150
10,220	2.92	2.92	152.92
20,440	5.84	8.76	158.76
30,660	8.76	17.52	167.52
40,880	11.68	29.20	179.20
51,100	14.60	43.80	193.80
61,320	17.52	61.32	211.32
71,540	20.44	81.76	231.76
81,760	23.36	105.12	255.12
91,980	26.28	131.40	281.40
102,200	29.20	160.60	310.60

As you can see, under these conditions, the pounds really start to add up as the years go by.

Of course, most of us who weigh 150 pounds at age 25 do not double our weight by the time we are 35. That is because most of us *do* eat less as the years go by.

But what these figures show is just how much less we must eat if we are to maintain our desired weight level.

The simple truth is that if we eat the same amount at age 35 as we did at age 25, we will gain 29 pounds in that year alone.

And, as we grow older, it only gets worse.

Luckily, our appetite gradually diminishes with age and most of us do cut down our food intake.

Unfortunately, most of us do not cut down *enough* and that is why more than half of the population of the United States is overweight.

What is amazing is how little you have to overeat to gain a lot of weight. Consider this: A pat of butter contains only 36 calories. If you overeat by only this much every day, in ten years you will gain 37½ pounds.

Now consider this: So far we have been talking about what happens to people who have a more or less *normal* metabolism. For these people the problem is even worse.

Fortunately, in many cases now it is possible to speed up a sluggish metabolism.

So hang in there. You'll soon learn just how to do this in the "Good News" section of this book. But right now please go on to Chapter IV where you will learn about another serious problem faced by all weight watchers.

CHAPTER IV

THE WORST ADDICTION IN THE WORLD

There are many addictions that are hard to break.

Millions of people have a hard time with alcohol. Millions more have tried to quit smoking and failed. There are hundreds of thousands of drug addicts who would give anything to be free of their chemical prisons.

But as terrible as these addictions are, there is one that is even harder to kick than all of the above put together.

It is overeating.

More than half of all adult Americans are overweight. Almost all of these people have gone on a diet of one kind or another in a desperate attempt to stop overeating. In the long run, almost 100% of them fail. Even those who do manage to lose some weight, usually regain every pound they have lost and more.

Actually, the cure rate of nicotine fiends, alcoholics, and drug addicts is higher than the cure rate of overeaters.

Let's say that you are a heavy smoker *and* an overeater and you have made up your mind to make an heroic effort to kick both habits.

You decide to quit smoking first and then tackle the overeating problem later on. You throw your cigarettes away. This is it. Cold turkey. The foul things will never touch your lips again.

Here's how it goes.

The first day is bad. All of a sudden you become aware of how many daily "events" trigger off your desire to smoke.

You want a cigarette every time you have a cup of coffee. Every time you finish eating. Whenever you have a drink. After making love. Before going to bed. As soon as you get up.

And so on.

The second and third day is even worse. You begin to suffer very real and unpleasant withdrawal symptoms. It is brutal. You are coming to understand that smoking is more than just a habit; it is an honest-to-God chemical addiction just like heroin or morphine.

But you grit your teeth and hold on. As the days go by, your desire to smoke gradually starts to lessen. Finally, after about three weeks, most of the residual nicotine has been flushed out of your body and you only crave a cigarette a few times a day.

Then one find day you wake up with a big smile and you realize that you haven't even *thought* about smoking for a whole week.

You've done it! You've kicked the habit! Now you

are ready to tackle your problem of overeating and that ought to be easy compared to what you've just been through. After all, smoking is an actual drug addiction and overeating is just a habit - right?

Well maybe. Let's see how it goes.

First of all, to get started, you pick out a nice healthy 1,200 calorie a day diet and you promise yourself to stay on it until all your extra pounds are gone.

Unlike when you quit smoking, the first day of your new diet is not so bad at all. And also, unlike cigarettes, you don't have to give up food altogether—you only have to cut down.

The next few days aren't bad either. You are excited about your new diet and the idea of looking good again and this more than offsets the minor inconvenience of being hungry once in awhile.

After about a week, however, it starts to get harder. The newness of the diet is wearing off and you are getting a little tired of being constantly hungry.

Oddly enough, at the same point in time where it got easier to stop smoking, it is getting harder to keep dieting.

But you are strong. You hang in there.

Unfortunately though, it gets harder and harder every day. It seems like you think about food all the time. Soon you notice that you are only living for the day you reach your desired weight level so you can go off your diet. The truth of the matter is that all you want to do is eat. You are literally consumed by thoughts of food.

And sooner or later after X number of days or X number of weeks, you just can't stand it any more and you go off your diet.

With a vengeance.

You eat and eat and eat. It's as though you can't help yourself. It seems like you are absolutely *driven* to make up for all that suffering you've just been through.

Soon, if you are like most people, you will have

gained back every single pound you have lost and more.

And also, if you are like most people, sooner or later you will once again be ashamed to be so fat and you will start looking around for another diet.

Probably, however, whatever new diet you find will most likely produce the same results.

That is because almost every diet on the market has the same major flaw. This major flaw makes almost certain that none of these diets can work for you in the long run.

You see, you can give up smoking and drugs and alcohol *completely!* Your body doesn't really need these substances. And it is a lot easier to give up smoking completely than it is to cut down to 5 or 6 cigarettes a day. The same is true of drugs and alcohol.

But you can't give up eating completely. You have to have food. And what happens on most diets is that you eat just enough to "tease" yourself and to wake up your hunger.

After awhile it becomes unbearable.

What is this flaw that all of these deals have in common? The answer is simple—*on all of these diets it gets harder every day!*

That's way it is often easier to quit smoking or stop drinking or even to rid yourself of an addiction to hard drugs than it is to diet. With smoking, alcohol, and drugs it gets *easier* as times goes by.

With dieting it is just the opposite. *It gets harder every day!* After awhile on most diets you are constantly hungry and you can't think about anything else but food.

If you have a lot of willpower, you might be able to endure this suffering for a few days or a few weeks (maybe even a few months) but your willpower just can't stand up to *constant* day in and day out hunger.

And even if you could endure this constant suffering - so what? What good is it to be thin if you are miserable and hungry all the time. What kind of a life is that?

What you really need is a diet strategy that breaks up this cycle of suffering. You need a plan that lets you get some fun out of life. A plan that sees to it that you are never hungry. A plan that lets you satisfy your desire for food so that you can think about something else once in awhile.

Is there such a plan? Is there such a plan that frees you from this gnawing "deprivation buildup?" A plan that lets you eat your cake and lose weight too?

Yes there is. In fact, there are easy answers to all three of the major problems I have described so far. And now that you have digested the bad news, please turn the page so we can cheer ourselves up with the good news we're about to learn.

CHAPTER V

THE MIRACLE OF FRUCTOSE

As we learned in Chapter II, the secret truth about fat people is that they are constantly hungry.

We also learned that this is often because of an abnormal insulin response to sugar in our diet.

This chapter is going to explain a way that you can sour sweet tooth and lose weight too. It will introduce you to a remarkable natural food substance called fructose which has some highly unique properties.

To make this chapter easier to understand and hopefully more entertaining, we're going to do it in a question and answer format. The questions are those that you might like to ask me in a face to face interview.

Here we go.

Q. What exactly is fructose?

A. Fructose is a natural sugar found in honey and certain fruits. It is commonly referred to as fruit sugar.

Q. What does it taste like?

A. It looks and tastes exactly like ordinary table sugar (sucrose) except that it is a little sweeter.

Q. Since it is sweeter, does it have more calories than regular sugar?

A. No. It has exactly the same—16 per teaspoonful.

Q. How do you use fructose?

A. You can use it just like you use ordinary sugar except you may want to use a little less because it is 1/3 sweeter.

Q. Since you don't have to use as much fructose to get the same sweetness as you would with regular sugar, won't that save a lot of calories?

A. Yes. If a recipe calls for 1 cup of sugar, you

only need 2/3 cup of a cup if you are using fructose. But saving calories is not the important thing about fructose.

Q. I don't understand. If saving calories is not the important thing then just what is the big deal about fructose?

A. The big deal about fructose is that when it enters your body, it has a very different effect on you than ordinary sugar.

Q. How so?

A. For one thing, it is more slowly absorbed into your bloodstream. For another, fructose is the only sugar that can be assimilated *directly* into your muscle cells. But the most important thing of all is that *fructose raises your blood sugar level without creating an insulin response!*

Q. Why is that so important?

A. Are you kidding? Just think about what that means! It means that from now on whenever you get hungry, you can eat or drink something sweet to raise your blood sugar level and bring your hunger to a dead full stop! *And* since your body won't be producing any insulin to pull that sugar right back out of your bloodstream—not only will your blood sugar level go up, it will *stay* up!

In other words—now, at last—you can eat or drink something sweet to satisfy your hunger and your hunger will *stay* satisfied.

Q. That sounds fantastic. Why haven't I heard about this before?

A. Actually, fructose has been widely used in Europe but it is just starting to catch on over here. After this book comes out, I'll bet that almost every weight watcher in the country will start to use it. It's already starting to catch on like wildfire here in Hollywood.

Q. This sounds almost too good to be true. Are you sure it is safe?

A. Yes, it is. Remember, this is a food, *not* a drug. In fact, if you are overweight, it is probably much better for your system than ordinary sugar because it does not induce an insulin response.

Q. There's gotta be something bad about it. Doesn't it have any drawbacks at all?

A. Well, there isn't any kind of sugar that is good for your teeth so be sure to brush three times a day. And, of course, if you are a diabetic you should check with your doctor before using *any kind* of sugar. You should also check with your doctor to make sure that fructose will not contribute to any triglyceride problem you might be developing.

Q. I'm not a diabetic and just for the record, I've been brushing three times a day for years. Is there anything else I should know?

A. Nothing bad. As a matter of fact, there are a couple more good things I haven't told you yet.

Q. Tell me. Tell me. I'm all ears. What are you waiting for?

A. Don't be so impatient. I'm doing the best I can. Anyway, two more good things about fructose are the way it relieves a hangover and the way it soothes jangled nerves.

Q. Wait a minute. Let's take these points one at a time. How in the world does fructose relieve a hangover?

A. If you drink too much, you will wake up tired and cranky. This is because your body has been using up so much energy to burn off all that extra alcohol. If you take some fructose at night before you go to bed and again as soon as you wake up, you will have a constant stream of energy that will keep you steady as a rock. There is a good article about this in the February 1978 edition of OUI magazine titled "Sometimes a Great Potion".

Q. That's fascinating. Of course, I'm not much of a drinker so tell me about how fructose calms your nerves.

A. There is a whole book written about this. It is called "Diet Away Your Stress, Tension and Anxiety." This book tells how the proper use of fructose in your diet can dramatacially reduce your tension level because it blocks what the authors call the stress response.

Q. How does this work?

A. It's a chemical thing and to tell you the truth it's a little bit complicated. If you want to know more, you can read the book. It is well researched and it is available in paperback. By the way, the reason it works may be complicated, but the results are simple. If you are nervous, fructose just plain calms you down. At least that's been the experience of a lot of people, including the authors of this book.

Q. Let me see if I've got this straight. Are you telling me that fructose will give me more energy, knock out my hunger, cure my hangovers and calm my nerves?

A. Yes.

Q. I gotta try this stuff. Where do I get it? How much does it cost? How do I use it? Do you have any fructose recipes? Can I just mix it up in my coffee? Can I...

A. Hold it! Have a little patience. You are going to learn the answers to all these questions and more a little later on. I will tell you that you can go to your local health food store and they'll have fructose on a shelf in granulated or tablet form. If they are out they can easily order it for you. It's more expensive than sugar but good things usually are.

Right now, however, it is important that you understand one more very important fact about losing weight. Please go on to the next chapter.

CHAPTER VI

TURNING UP THE FURNACE

As we learned in Chapter III, a sluggish metabolism can cause real problems for dieters. This chapter will try to give you some help with that problem.

It is your thyroid gland that regulates your metabolism.

This is one of the larger glands in your body and it is located in your neck right in front of your windpipe.

If your thyroid gland was seriously *overactive,* your emotions would become greatly exaggerated and your behavior would follow suit.

If your thyroid gland stopped working altogether, your IQ would drop to the level of a three year old child.

All of the above conditions are medical problems and far beyond the scope of this book.

What we are concerned with here is what happens if your thyroid is just a *little bit underactive.*

If this is the case, then your metabolism will be slightly lower than it should be and we already know what that means.

Very simply, it means that some of the food you eat every day that would normally be converted to energy will, instead, be stored in your body as a fat deposit.

And, of course, as we have seen in the last chapter, these fat deposits can add up to a massive weight gain in a relatively short period of time.

Your thyroid gland needs iodine to function properly. Years ago, it was fairly common to see such an enlargement of the thyroid gland which resulted in a swelling in the front of the neck. For those of you who are too young to remember, this was commonly referred to as a goiter.

After we started putting iodine into our salt, this problem pretty much disappeared.

It is true that if you consume a lot of salt that you will probably get enough iodine for your thyroid to function properly.

However, for people who need to lose weight, this creates another problem.

Namely—water retention.

If you eat too much salt (and most people eat way too much), your body will become waterlogged.

This will give you a bloated look and add to your weight problem.

By the way, did you know that many people can lose as much as eight pounds simply by eliminating salt from their diet?

It's true. Anyway, the problem for dieters is to cut down or eliminate salt and at the same time make sure that the thyroid gets enough iodine to function properly.

There is an easy way to do this.

All you have to do is add kelp to your diet. Kelp is the best source of organic iodine. It is a natural salt substitute made from certain seaweeds. It also contains calcium, potassium and various trace minerals in addition to iodine.

Granular kelp is available in any good health food store and many regular supermarkets.

If you will add just one teaspoon of kelp to your diet every day, your thyroid should have all the iodine it needs to function properly.

If, at the same time, you eliminate salt from your diet, you will get a double benefit. The kelp can help wake up a "sleepy" thyroid gland and increase the amount of calories your body burns each day. This, of course, allows you to eat more without a weight gain.

And by eliminating salt you will give your body a chance to throw off the excess water you have been carrying around.

You can't lose. You win both ways.

In case you are wondering, kelp is quite tasty and many people like it better than salt. You can keep it in a shaker just like salt and use it on whatever food you wish to season.

The only thing that takes some getting used to is asking people to "pass the kelp shaker, please."

Whatever you do, make sure you get enough iodine.

Adele Davis, the world famous nutritionist, has written that all sick people, all people with high blood pressure, *and all overweight people* need *extra* iodine.

Take her word for it. She's right.

Now let's go to the next chapter for a solution to another problem.

CHAPTER VII

BREAKING UP THE CYCLE OF SUFFERING

In Chapter IV we discussed the reasons why overeating is the most difficult addiction in the world to overcome.

We learned that when someone is trying to give up nicotine, alcohol or drugs, that every day he or she is able to hang in there, it gets easier. We also learned that when we try to rid ourselves of the habit of overeating, that it works just the opposite way. In other words, when we diet, it gets harder every day.

In this chapter, I am going to tell you about a very simple technique that will effectively break up this cycle of misery. This simple technique will make it possible for you to stay on this or literally any diet for the rest of your life.

Most people when they go on a diet, do so with the idea that they will remain on the diet for a certain period of time and/or until they have lost a certain amount of weight. At the end of that time period, they plan on going off the diet and eating more or less regularly so as to maintain their weight loss. Well, that might be the plan but in fact that is not the way it usually works out. Instead, what usually happens is that after so many days or so many weeks of suffering, the poor dieter goes off his diet and eats in anything but a normal fashion. What he does is eat and eat in an effort to make up for all of that misery he has endured.

Since this strategy is almost certain to fail, what we need to lose weight successfully is a brand new strategy. And here it is: Instead of dieting every day, *we are going to diet only every other day!*

That sounds very simple, doesn't it? Actually, it is a very simple idea but it also is a very important one.

You see, contrary to popular opinion, many overweight people have much more willpower than thin people when it comes to dieting. Most overweight people would find it a snap to eat virtually nothing or to go on an extremely strict diet if they only had to do so for one day. As a matter of fact, most overweight people have gone on several near starvation diets for days or weeks on end before their willpower finally caved in.

But think of this—with the every other day idea, you only have to suffer "one day at a time". That will be a snap for most dieters. After all, it would be very easy to eat little or nothing on Monday if you knew you could eat pretty much whatever you wished on Tuesday. Would it not?

Of course it would. And not only that, since you are going to be using fructose to curb your hunger, you won't even have to "suffer" much on your diet days.

You see, this way you can diet on Monday and then eat normally on Tuesday and then diet again Wednesday and eat normally on Thursday and so on, without the buildup of suffering that accumulates whenever you try the normal method of dieting every day.

I know that this is an extremely simple idea. But sometimes the simplest ideas are the very best. I can tell you that this idea has made all the difference in the world to me.

When I was more than 40 pounds overweight, the idea of never eating enough to satisfy my hunger until I had lost the entire 40 pounds was like asking somebody to run a thousand miles without a moment's rest. But when I discovered that I could diet one day and eat normally the next day, it became very easy. This way I don't have to walk around feeling deprived and left out all the time. If I get a little uncomfortable on whatever day I happen to be dieting, I can console myself with the knowledge that as soon as I go to bed and wake up in the morning, I can eat normally. And I have found out that I can handle almost anything one day at a time.

So far in this book you have learned all about what I consider to be the three major obstacles to successful dieting and also you have learned how to overcome these obstacles. The ideas presented in this and the previous two chapters will constitute your major artillery in the war against fat. However, there are some other important weapons in the fight against fat that you should know about.

That's what the next chapter is all about.

CHAPTER VIII

SOME ADDITIONAL WEAPONS

The idea behind this chapter is to make you aware of some of the weapons you have available to you in your fight against fat. Many of these weapons are totally unknown to 99% of the general public. Many of these ideas are quite unconventional, but all of them can help you in your never ending struggle to stay slim.

THE MAGIC NO-HUNGER MILKSHAKE

Put 1 1/2 glasses of skim milk into a blender. Then add: 1 tbsp. safflower oil, 1 tbsp. fructose, 1 tsp. vanilla extract. Now start your blender on low and add: 1 tbsp. powdered brewer's yeast, 1 tbsp. lecithin, 1 tsp. granulated kelp.

This milkshake offers a number of benefits to anyone who is struggling to lose weight. First of all the fructose and powdered brewer's yeast and skim milk are three of the most potent hunger fighters known to man. I think it would be very unusual for anyone to drink this milkshake and be hungry at all for at least three hours. The safflower oil will help flush the excess water from your body and the kelp may help to raise the efficiency of your metabolism. The lecithin in the milkshake is a powerful nerve nutrient and with the fructose can create a remarkable calming effect. This is especially helpful if you have trouble with insomnia. Taken just before bedtime, this magic milkshake can act as an organic sleeping pill and actually help you lose weight while you sleep. Lecithin also will help to dissolve and break up fat globules in your body so that they may be more easily flushed from your system. The powdered brewer's yeast contains more concentrated B vitamins than any other food in nature. B vitamins are especially helpful in times of stress and, of course, any time you are dieting it does create some stress.

So all in all, this milkshake is a wonderful boon for dieters. It can stop your hunger, calm your nerves and be a great help in overcoming stress.

SIX LIQUID WILLPOWER NO-HUNGER DRINKS

All of these liquid willpower no-hunger drinks contain fructose. Essentially, that is the secret of their effectiveness.

Actually, there are probably several hundred ways of mixing fructose with different liquids in order to form an effective no-hunger potion. However, what I am attempting to do here is to give you a few ideas that have worked for me and then perhaps you may want to go on to experiment on your own.

1. *Grapefruit juice and fructose*

All you do is take an 8 oz. glass of grapefruit juice and add 1-2 tsp. of fructose. Grapefruit juice is a natural hunger fighter by itself and with the fructose, it becomes an easily made but quite powerful hunger fighter.

2. *Coffee and fructose*

All you do here is substitute for table sugar in your coffee. Coffee has a tendency to depress your appetite a little bit by itself and the fructose, of course, makes it just that much more effective.

3. *Fructose lemonade*

Simply squeeze the juice of half a lemon into a glass of water and add a couple of teaspoons of fructose. This is my personal favorite. It is fast and easy to make. It is delicious and satisfying. I generally can count upon it stopping my hunger for an hour or two.

4. *Herb tea and fructose*

Certain herb teas have a tranquilizing effect on your nervous system. This seems to be especially true of camomile tea. Therefore, one of my favorite no-hunger drinks, when I am tense, is camomile tea with 2 tsp. of fructose. If you are jittery, I think you will especially like this one.

5. *Warm milk and fructose*

Sometimes I like to use this just before I go to bed. The warm milk and the fructose act together as a natural sleeping pill for me. Also, I have found it is difficult for me to go to bed hungry and this wonderful concoction eliminates that discomfort.

6. *Tonic water and fructose*

This makes a good substitution for

cocktails at your next party. Include a couple of ice cubes and a slice of lemon and it looks exactly like you're having a gin and tonic.

Now, of course, these are just ideas. I encourage you to experment. The amount of fructose you use in the various drinks does not have to be a fixed thing. Some people have found that they need a full tablespoon of fructose to effectively knock out their hunger, while others have found that they need as little as one teaspoon. Everyone is different. So as I said, experiment a little and find out what works for you.

THE WATERMELON FLUSH

Paul Bragg was one of the most knowledgeable men in the world on the subjects of diet and health. He was extremely active right up until his death recently at the ripe old age of 96.

One of his favorite diet secrets was the watermelon flush that he described in his books. This technique has a remarkable cleansing effect on the body and provides an amazingly fast weight loss.

All that you need do to get these benefits is simply to eat nothing but watermelon for an entire day. You can have as much as you like, but don't have anything else.

When you weigh yourself the next morning, you may very well be astonished at how much weight you've lost. You will also probably be calmer and more clear headed than you have been for a long time.

Give it a try. It's easy and it works.

THE PAPAYA PURGE

A friend of mine who has been around the Hollywood scene for quite some time told me about this one. It seems that whenever certain Indian yogis are desirous of a fast weight loss, they eat nothing but papayas for a day or so.

I tried it and it works. In fact, I personally lose

more weight eating my fill of papayas than I do on a complete water fast. Perhaps this is so because of the laxative and diuretic effects of this delicious fruit.

By the way, mangoes work too and some people like them better.

EAT BEFORE YOU EAT

Most people don't know it, but it takes about 20 minutes after you start eating for your blood sugar to rise high enough for your body to stop sending hunger signals.

Quite often we can eat enough to satisfy our *true* hunger in the first five minutes of a meal. However, we may not realize that it is time to stop eating for another full 15 minutes, and if you are anything like me, you can eat an enormous amount in those 15 minutes.

Luckily there is an easy solution to this problem. All you have to do is eat before you eat. In other words, simply have a small snack about 20 minutes before you sit down to the table. This will do just what your mommy said it would—it will ruin your appetite. This is especially true if you eat or drink something that contains fructose.

I know this is a simple idea but it can be a real diet saver. It will help you take the edge off your hunger and help you avoid hysterical overeating.

LECITHIN

Lecithin is a remarkable food substance available at any good health food store. It has the property of liquifying fat and globules and thereby enabling them to be more readily flushed out of the body. Lecithin is also an excellent nerve nutrient and it helps promote a sense of well-being. A recent article in a large newspaper told of research by a team of medical professionals that indicates that eating lecithin can increase your intelligence by as much as 25 percent. I can't vouch for that. I can't promise that lecithin will make you smarter but I can promise that it will help you in your efforts to lose weight.

BREWER'S YEAST

I know I have already mentioned lecithin and brewer's yeast when I gave you the recipe for my magic no-hunger milkshake, but both of these ingredients are important diet aids and that's why I've chosen to elaborate on them here.

Powdered brewer's yeast is probably the most highly concentrated protein food found in nature. It is also nature's most complete form of B vitamins. It contains almost no fat and the concentrated protein seems to work like powdered heat. It seems to activate your body's inner furnace to break down stubborn fat.

I strongly suggest that you get into the habit of including this "wonder food" in your daily diet.

Now let's go on to Chapter IX where we shall put everything you have learned so far into a basic plan of attack in our war against unsightly fat.

CHAPTER IX

SUMMARY AND PLAN OF ATTACK

By now, you know more about the real problems of dieting than perhaps 99% of the people in this country.

You have taken in a lot of valuable information. Before we go on to the actual step-by-step mechanics of the diet, let's review what you have learned so far and put it all together in a basic plan of attack.

Here are some of the important facts we have covered.

FACT: On the average, our metabolism decreases about one percent per year after age 25 and this one percent a year decrease can add up to a massive weight gain if we are not careful.

FACT: We can help make sure that our metabolism is up to par by adding kelp to our diet on a daily basis as this insures that our thyroid is getting enough iodine to function properly.

FACT: Salt causes us to retain excess water and using kelp as a salt substitute can eliminate this problem.

FACT: The secret truth about fat people is that they are often hungry because their bodies tend to produce too much insulin and this causes a low blood sugar condition which triggers off hunger signals.

FACT: We can at least partially alleviate this hyperinsulinism condition by substituting fructose for sucrose and eliminating starchy foods from our diets.

FACT: It is almost impossible to stay on any weight loss diet day in and day out without a letup. This is because of a factor we call "deprivation buildup."

FACT: We can overcome "deprivation buildup" by dieting only every other day.

FACT: Dieting is a stress and apt to make us irritable.

FACT: We can help alleviate the stress of dieting by adding certain "nerve nutrient" foods to our meals.

FACT: It takes about twenty minutes for our blood sugar to rise after we start to eat. This means that if we eat enough to satisfy our hunger in the first five minutes of our meal, we may not know it for another fifteen minutes and as a result, we may overeat during the remaining fifteen minutes.

FACT: We can raise our blood sugar level before we sit down to a meal by simply snacking on something about twenty minutes before meal time. This will tend to take the edge off our hunger and make us much less likely to overeat.

FACT: One of the fastest and easiest ways to lose weight in a 24-hour period is to eat nothing but watermelon.

FACT: Another extremely fast and easy way to lose weight in a 24-hour period is to eat nothing but papayas.

FACT: And yet another way is to eat nothing but mangoes. So now we come to our basic plan of attack. Here is what we are going to do.

1. We are only going to diet every other day.
2. We are going to stop using sucrose and start using fructose.
3. We are going to make use of the unique

properties of watermelons, papayas and mangoes to speed our slimming efforts.
4. We are going to stop using salt and start using kelp.
5. We are going to start adding "nerve nutrient" foods to our diet to help fight the stress of dieting and living in general.
6. We are going to start eliminating refined starches from our diets.
7. We are *not* going to count calories or grams of carbohydrates. The only thing we are going to keep track of is our daily weight loss.

This then is our basic plan of attack. In the next chapter we will start getting more specific as we examine exactly what we will be eating on our "diet days."

CHAPTER X

DIET DAYS

Here are 14 different day ideas.

You can use a different one each new diet day or you can use the same one over and over.

1. *Fruit Juice* - That's it. Nothing else. No solid food at all. You can have up to six (but not more) 8-ounce glasses of any kind of fruit juice you prefer. Fresh juice is best. If you must use canned juice, make sure no sugar or artificial sweetners have been added. Use only one kind of juice all day. However, you can use a different juice on each new diet day.

2. *Eggs and Tomatoes* - This is a California favorite. All you have all day is six eggs and six tomatoes. The eggs can be boiled or poached or fried in a teflon skillet. For seasoning you can use kelp and pepper. No salt.

3. *Fruit only* - What could be simpler? Choose any fruit you like but stay with the same one all day. You can have up to six pieces.

4. *Health Milk Shake* - Whomp it up according to the directions in Chapter VIII and sip it all day as the mood moves you.

5. *Watermelon* - My favorite. Eat all you want, but remember - no salt.

6. *Mangoes* - Nothing else but you may have all you want.

7. *Papayas* - Ditto.

8. *Total Fasting* - Nothing but water all day. Preferably bottled spring or distilled.

9. *Bananas and Skim Milk Shake* - Mix up one banana and a glass of skim milk in your blender to

make a creamy shake and drink it down. Enjoy. You can do this three times a day.

10. *Ice Cream* - You can have three cups of any flavor you choose. Who says dieting has to be wretched.

11. *Yogurt* - Same as above. Three cups of any flavor you choose.

12. *Boiled Eggs and Oranges* - Six boiled eggs and three fresh oranges. Space them out over the day. No salt on the eggs. Use kelp and pepper instead.

13. *Salad and Fish* - Here you can have a green salad with Italian (vinegar and oil) dressing and six ounces of broiled fish seasoned with pepper, kelp and lemon juice three times a day.

14. *Three Small Balanced Meals* - This is the most conventional of the lot. You can plan the meals but make sure you are true to yourself and that the meals are indeed small enough to insure a loss.

At this point don't worry if these diet day ideas seem severe to you. Remember, you get to eat normally again the *very next day!*

By the way, on your diet days, you should be sure to take one tablespoon of fructose with a no-calorie beverage whenever you *first start* to get hungry.

This should keep your energy level up and your hunger level down all day.

Now let's go on to the next chapter and talk about your eating days.

CHAPTER XI

EATING DAYS

Your eating days are much more flexible than your diet days.

You can make up your own meal plans and eat a wide variety of foods so long as you follow the following rules.

DO: Have one teaspoon of fructose in a no-calorie beverage twenty minutes before every meal. Have one teaspoon of fructose in a no-calorie beverage anytime you *first start* to get hungry.

Add at least one teaspoon of granular kelp to your diet every day.

Learn to listen to your body and stop eating when you are no longer hungry.

Start adding "nerve nutrient" foods to your meals.

DON'T: Eat regular sugar (sucrose) or anything made with sucrose—be careful here. Sugar is hidden in almost everything. Check labels carefully. Remember, fructose will not curb your hunger if you continue to eat sucrose.

DON'T: Eat anything made with white flour. White flour is quickly converted to sugar (not fructose) after it enters your system. This, of course, will create an insulin response.

DON'T: Add salt to your food. It is also a good idea to avoid foods that are already salted. In any case, for sure don't use any salt from the shaker.

You can easily observe the above rules and at the same time have an endless variety of healthful and satisfying meals. Here are three examples of typical eating days:

Breakfast	Have a teaspoonful of fructose with coffee or tea twenty minutes before eating.
	One-half cantaloupe
	Two eggs
	Whole wheat toast and butter
Lunch	Bowl of soup
	Rye Krisp crackers
	Milk
	Apple
Dinner	Salad with two tablespoons dressing
	Steak
	Baked potato with butter
	Broccoli
Snack	Popcorn
	Coffee

Breakfast	Bowl of cereal with skim milk, fructose and banana
	Orange juice
Lunch	Tuna sandwich on whole wheat bread
	Cucumbers and tomatoes
	Coffee or tea
Dinner	Baked chicken
	Corn on the cob
	Large salad with dressing
Snack	Celery stuffed with peanut butter
Breakfast	Cheese omelette
	Whole wheat English muffin
	Tomato Juice
Lunch	Hamburger on whole wheat bun
	French fries
Dinner	Fish seasoned with butter
	Large salad with dressing
	Green beans
	Strawberries sprinkled with fructose

As you can see, your eating days can be varied, satisfying and enjoyable.

Some people find it hard to believe that you can eat this much and still lose weight. But you can! The key, of course, is that your "diet days" are quite stringent.

And also, of course, it is easy to tolerate your diet days because you can look forward to eating your fill the very next day.

Actually, with the help of fructose, even your diet days will be quite painless.

Now let's go on to the next chapter and pull everything together in a specific step-by-step plan.

CHAPTER XII

PUTTING IT TOGETHER STEP-BY STEP

This will be a short chapter as the mechanics of this diet are remarkably simple. Here are the steps.

Step 1 -   Visit your doctor and explain the diet to him and get his OK.

Step 2 -   *First day.* Start your diet with a watermelon flush. As you will recall from Chapter VIII, this means that you will eat nothing but watermelon for an entire day. You can, however, have as much as you want and you can continue to drink no-calorie beverages such as coffee or tea. (This will be a surprisingly easy and satisfy-day for you.)

Step 3 - *Second day*. Follow the rules given in Chapter XI and have yourself a satisfying "eating day."

Step 4 - *Third day*. Pick a diet day idea from Chapter X and stick with it all day.

Step 5 - Repeat steps 3 and 4 until you reach your desired weight. That's it. That is all there is to it. It is really just that simple. You simply start your diet with a watermelon flush and then alternate diet days with eating days until you have reached your desired weight level.

Remember to keep a supply of fructose on hand and have some whenever you *first start to get hungry*. Also remember to "eat before you eat" on your eating days.

If you would like to help us with our continuing research, you can fill in the forms on the next few pages which charts your progress for the first thirty-one days. We would especially appreciate your comments and suggestions.

In any case, since most people who go on a diet want to look as good as possible, we think you will enjoy the next chapter titled "The Greatest Beauty Secret in the World."

NOTE

Fill in this part
of form before
starting diet.

Age _____ Date _____

Height _____ *Morning Weight _____

Bust _____ Waist _____

Hips _____

*Weigh yourself right after you get up and after using the bathroom and before you get dressed.

DAILY PROGRESS RECORD

Fill in this part
of form daily for
the first 31 days

                                      Morning Weight

Day 1	Watermelon flush	_____
Day 2	Eating day	_____
Day 3	Diet day	_____
Day 4	Eating day	_____
Day 5	Diet day	_____
Day 6	Eating day	_____
Day 7	Diet day	_____
Day 8	Eating day	_____
Day 9	Diet day	_____
Day 10	Eating day	_____
Day 11	Diet day	_____
Day 12	Eating Day	_____
Day 13	Diet day	_____
Day 14	Eating day	_____
Day 15	Diet day	_____
Day 16	Eating day	_____
Day 17	Diet day	_____

Fill in this part
of form daily for
the first 31 days

Day 18   Eating day   _____
Day 19   Diet day   _____
Day 20   Eating day   _____
Day 21   Diet day   _____
Day 22   Eating day   _____
Day 23   Diet day   _____
Day 24   Eating day   _____
Day 25   Diet day   _____
Day 26   Eating day   _____
Day 27   Diet day   _____
Day 28   Eating day   _____
Day 29   Diet day   _____
Day 30   Eating day   _____
Day 31   Diet day   _____

Note

Fill in this part
of the form after
you have been on the diet for 31 days.

Age _____ Date _____
Height _____ *Morning Weight _____
Bust _____ Waist _____
Hips _____

*Weigh yourself right after you get up and after using the bathroom and before you get dressed.

After you have completed these forms, please mail to:

    Millburn Book Corporation

    P.O. Box 1013

    343 Millburn Avenue

    Millburn, New Jersey 07041

Comments _____
    or   _____
Suggestions _____

CHAPTER XIII

THE GREATEST BEAUTY SECRET IN THE WORLD

I am going to reveal to you in this chapter what I consider to be not only the greatest beauty secret in the world, but also perhaps the greatest health secret in the world.

In Chapter III, we talked about how our metabolism decreases approximately 1% a year after the age of 25. And how this slight decrease can add up to a massive weight gain over the years. We learned that if our metabolism is not high enough to burn up all of the food we eat, that the excess will be stored in our bodies as fat.

But in this day and age, all of us consume a lot more than food. Nowadays, we take into our bodies several hundred unnatural chemicals and chemical compounds each day. Many of these unnatural chemicals are metabolized out of our bodies. However, as our metabolism decreases, we are unable to handle these chemicals and other impurities the way we could when we were younger.

The result? Some of these chemicals and impurities consumed have to be stored in our bodies along with that part of our food we are unable to metabolize completely. What happens is that since our bodies cannot burn up all of this "sludge," we have to store it some place and we store it inside each of our cells, within our body organs, in our skin, on the inside of our blood vessels, and practically everywhere throughout our bodies.

Our bodies are comprised of billions and billions of cells. If we are unable to metabolize all we consume, the excess is stored in each of our individual cells. Try to imagine an individual cell as a small sponge. Now imagine that each of these small sponges is soaked and saturated with various impurities and unnatural chemical compounds. All of our "sponges" become clogged as we grow older because our decreased metabolism does not provide the vitality to burn off the impurities.

As a result, our cells are clogged up and unclean and if examined under a microscope, would no longer have the clean, fresh appearance of a new cell. Since everything in your body is made up of cells, you can only look as bright and shiny and clean and clear as the condition of your cells permit. In other words, if you want to look as good as possible, what you really have to do is flush out the impurities and unnatural chemical compounds from each of the billions of cells in your body.

Once you learn how to do this, the results can be truly amazing. Your skin will soften and clear up. Your eyes will take a new shine. Your hair will become more lustrous. And in general, you will have a fresh, scrubbed, clear, clean look about you that most people have not enjoyed since their early 20's or even perhaps their teens.

Needless to say, many of the people here in Hollywood who must look their best at all times, have learned the secret of keeping their bodies more or less free of impurities, and thus enabling them to have the appearance of youth.

There are many health and beauty secrets used by people in Hollywood, but I believe *the most valuable and powerful beauty and health tool of all is periodic fasting.*

If you have ever fasted, you already know the amazing results that can be obtained from even a short fast. If you have not, you are in for a pleasant surprise.

When you fast, you don't eat anything at all. All you consume is water, preferably distilled or mineral, or fresh fruit juices. Here is what happens when you fast: First of all, since you are not consuming any food, this gives your overworked metabolism and digestive functions a chance to burn off all of the impurities that have been accumulating in your body over the years. It is, in fact, a sort of housecleaning. Also during a fast, your metabolism is stepped up. As the impurities begin to leave your body, you can actually see it by looking at your tongue. Your tongue will become coated and your breath will become foul. This is a good sign. It is, in fact, a sign that the impurities and unnatural chemicals are being flushed out of your body.

You should not attempt to take a long fast without

medical supervision. However, after checking with your doctor, you will probably find it beneficial to get into the habit of taking short, periodic fasts. For example, many people here in Hollywood make it a rule to fast every Monday. This enables them to set aside one day a week to cleanse their bodies and also allows them to live it up a little bit more on the other six days of the week without worrying too much about it.

Unless you are under supervision, you probably should never fast more than four days at any one time. It takes about four days to eliminate all of the salt, and therefore all the excess water from your body. A four-day fast can achieve remarkable results.

If you have never fasted, I would go so far as to say that in all probability, a four-day water fast will take as much as ten years off your appearance.

If you are new to fasting, it might sound like torture to you. However, you will be pleased to learn that fasting is perhaps the easiest of all ways to lose weight. This is because shortly after you go on a fast, your body begins to produce ketones which are natural appetite suppressors. Many people find it easier to fast than to tease themselves with a low calorie diet.

By the way, when you get into the habit of periodic fasting, you will not only be dramatically improving your appearance, you will also be dramatically improving your health. In short, what a fast does is give your body a chance to do some internal housecleaning and flush out the impurities that are stored in your arteries and tissues and vital organs. Naturally, this is not only good for your appearance, but it is also good for your all around general health.

Before you go on a fast of even one day, as a matter of fact, before you begin following the diet ideas in this book or any book, you should, of course, check with your doctor. If you get his OK, I would recommend that you begin by fasting one day every week. I like Mondays best. It gets my week off to a good start and it makes me feel sort of holy.

There isn't really a lot to know about the mechanics of fasting. All you do is stop eating. When I fast, I have nothing but distilled or mineral water. Other people prefer to drink fruit juices. Fruit jucies will work nearly as well as plain water. They just work a little slower.

After you have fasted one day a week for a few weeks, you may then want to try a four-day fast. I predict that after your first four-day fast, you will not believe the change in the way you feel and the change in the way you look.

An occasional day of fasting can be used as a substitute for your other diet day routines.

Many of the well known stars here in Hollywood have been fasting periodically for decades. I hope you are encouraged enough to check with your doctor and then give it a try.

CHAPTER XIV

HINTS FROM HOLLYWOOD

This chapter is simply a potpourri of diet and beauty ideas that I came across while researching this book. They are not written here in any particular order. I have merely set them down as they came to mind. Most of the ideas are quite unique and many of them are amazingly helpful. I suggest that you experiment a little and try out the ones that look good to you. You may very well be surprised at the results.

Three Reasons Not to Count Calories

1. It's boring. It takes up a lot of time and the people around you will justifiably grow tired of your fanaticism.

2. If you count calories, you will always be aware that you are on a diet. This then may occupy your mind so much you may be unable to concentrate on and find pleasure in other areas of your life. If you follow the diet recommendations in this book, you can lose weight without ever counting calories again.

3. Even if you do religiously attempt to keep track of your calories, you will probably miscount anyway. After all, can you tell the difference between a medium size apple and one a little larger than medium? And who in the world can figure out the calories involved in certain food combinations, such as sauces and casseroles? And if you underestimate your caloric intake by only fifty calories a day, you could gain as much as fifty pounds in a period of ten years. For the most part, all of this adds up to just one thing—counting calories just doen't work.

How Hollywood Stars Stop the Aging Process

The secret to remaining young is really quite simple. What you have to do is to stay healthy. Most of the signs of the so-called old age are really nothing more than signs of deteriorating health. If you look after your health—really look after it, you can retain the look and feel of youth well into your later years. Many of the stars who have been around for decades and still look trim and youthful regard their health as their most precious asset and they take very good care of that asset indeed.

There are many elements of health but below I am listing those that I feel are of particular importance because they are often overlooked.

The Seven Best Health Secrets of the Hollywood Stars

1. *Periodic Fasting* - I don't think I have to say more about this subject since it was all explained in Chapter XIII. However, I would like to reemphasize

that I consider "periodic fasting" to be the greatest health and beauty secret of all!

2. *Systematic Undereating* - You will find that most people who enjoy really excellent health, eat considerably less than is considered "normal." It has been estimated that Americans, on the average, eat *three times* as much as is needed to maintain health and vigor. I am sure you have heard the phrase "overfed and undernourished." This condition exists because when we eat too much our digestive system becomes so clogged that it cannot properly extract the nourishment from our food intake. When you systematically eat less, your digestive system has a chance to extract more of the nutrients from your food and thus do a more thorough job. Therefore, people who eat sparingly are often better nourished than those who make it a practice to gobble up everything in sight.

3. *Sweat* - It may sound funny, but the plain truth is that you just can't be really healthy unless you sweat a little every day. I understand that more than 60% of the toxins in our bodies are eliminated through our skin. Sweating is the principal way our skin throws off our accumulated waste and poisons. As I said in the last chapter, if you do not systematically eliminate the impurities in your system, they will build up and accumulate and eventually cause you grief. If you will work or exercise enough every day to work up a good sweat, not only will your health improve, but the quality of your skin improve dramatically.

4. *Enthusiasm* - Nearly everyone who lives a long time enjoys his life. Look at Bob Hope, he is in his mid-seventies and he looks like he is in his forties. He has the energy of a teenager. One of the reasons for his good health and boundless energy is simply that

he is in love with his life. If your life is dull and boring, try to find some way to liven it up. Get a more exciting job, try out a new hobby, start flirting more with the opposite sex. Do anything! But don't just sit there and vegetate!

5. *Romance* - Did you know that studies have shown that people who live past 100 have unusually active romance and sex lives? It's true, and scientists believe that this is one of the main factors that keeps them young. The message is clear - if you want to live a long time, you had better liven up your love life.

6. *Just Plain Fun* - It is amazing how many people get very little fun out of life. Actually, if you don't have fun, what is the point of living a long life anyway? I have noticed that most of the people who are chronologically old but biologically young seem to have an enormous amount of plain old-fashioned fun.

7. *A Good Doctor* - There is a night and day difference between doctors. You don't want a doctor who can simply help you when you are sick. What you need is a doctor who can teach you how to be extraordinarily well. I have my own criteria for identifying such doctors. What I look for is a doctor who is obviously in extra good physical shape himself. I wouldn't think of trusting my health to a doctor who smokes excessively, who is overweight and who breathes hard just walking around his office. And believe me, there are plenty of unhealthy doctors who don't know the first thing about nutrition or preventative health. In fact, did you know that the average age of a surgeon at death is only fifty-three? However, there are plenty of good doctors around and it is well worth your while to seek them out.

A Simple Five Second Exercise That Will Help You Get Rid of a Double Chin

Here's the way it works. Close your mouth and press the fingers of your left hand firmly into the area under your chin. Then press your tongue against the top of your mouth. If you do it correctly, you will feel the flesh under your chin tighten against your fingers. Hold this pressure for about five seconds and do it several times a day. After a few weeks you should notice a definite improvement in the muscle tone of this area.

How to Look Thin Before You Are Thin

You can appear to take off as much as ten pounds in ten minutes simply by choosing your clothes carefully. Many actresses are especially adept at wearing clothes that create the optical illusion of making them look like they have recently lost weight. Here are a few tricks that will help you achieve the same effect:

First of all, you should wear clothing that creates the illusion of length. Men will look slimmer if they wear a jacket and pants that are the same color and the illusion will be heightened if the shirt is also of the same color. What this does is create the impression of one long thinning flow of color. Women look slimmer when they wear deep or V necklines and simple and uncluttered styles. Lapels should be narrow and hemlines should be below the knee. It is best to wear soft fabrics that move with the body.

Dark colors are best. Wearing white, for example, can make you look up to ten pounds *heavier!* After you finish dressing, check yourself out in the mirror. As much as possible, what you want to achieve is the effect of one long flowing line from head to toe.

Anything that breaks the flow of this line, such as belts or boots or short skirts or even unnecessary jewelry and ornaments will have the opposite effect and make you look heavier.

A Certain Law You Must Obey For Every Pound You Take Off if You Want to Keep it Off

Here is the law: For every pound of fat you remove from your body, you must add a pound of excitement to your life. Believe it or not, a dieter's biggest problem is not hunger, it is boredom. If you lose a lot of weight and do not put more excitement into your life, it will be like getting all dressed up without having any place to go. Eventually, you will become bored so that even if you are not hungry, you will eat simply to relieve the boredom. Obey this law—it is not a small thing.

Why You Can Lose More Weight on This Diet Than if You Ran Seventy Miles Per Week

Most people don't know it but you only use approximately one hundred calories when you run a mile. Studies have shown also that it doesn't matter much how fast you run. A slow jog or a fast trot causes you to use approximately the same amount of calories. Therefore, if you ran as much as seventy miles per week, you would only be using up approximately 7,000 calories and 7,000 calories equals less than two pounds of fat. Needless to say, on the diet plan outlined in this book, you should lose considerably more than two pounds a week.

Six Foods That Give You an Emotional Lift

1. *Fructose* - We've talked a lot about fructose so far in this book but one thing I haven't mentioned is

that many people have told me that about ten minutes after they have taken a tablespoon of fructose they get a nice little buzz that makes them feel calm and confident. It doesn't happen to everybody but it does happen to some people, including the author.

2. *Brewer's Yeast* - We have talked about brewer's yeast before in this book and how it is chock full of B vitamins. If you have a B vitamin deficiency you may very well find that a daily ingestion of brewer's yeast will correct this situation and make you feel much better.

3. *Lecithin* - Lecithin is another one of those natural food substances that nourishes your nerves and if you are nervous and irritable normally, you may find that lecithin helps to promote a nice peaceful, easy feeling.

4. *Foods High in Calcium* - I didn't know it before I started researching this book but some nutritionists claim that calcium is one of the best pain fighters known to man. Apparently, calcium is one of the best substances you can ingest to relieve the pain of pleurisy, for example. And naturally, any time you relieve pain, you feel considerably better.

5. *Wheat Germ* - Sometimes wheat germ can make you feel better for the same reason that yeast does, namely, that it is also chock full of B vitamins. It tastes a lot better, too.

6. *Apple Cider Vinegar* - Anything that supplies you with nutrients of which you are deficient can make you feel better and many people are deficient in the minerals which are abundantly supplied in apple cidar vinegar.

How to Let Nature Give You a Natural Face Lift While You Sleep

This requires the use of a slant board. You can make one yourself or buy one inexpensively in many stores. The important thing is your feet being about three feet higher in elevation than your head. Here's how one woman uses the slant board: What she does is keep it beside her bed and when she wakes up in the morning, she gets out of bed, lays on the slant board and sleeps for another forty-five minutes. Thus the effects of gravity on her face are reversed and this tends to keep her face tight and youthful. It also has beneficial effects upon all the other parts of your body.

By the way, I would welcome any suggestions you might have that would be suitable for inclusion in this chapter in later editions of this book.

CHAPTER XV

GETTING INTO YOUR NEW ROLE

Now you know all of my diet secrets. You know how to strip the fat off of your body and you know how to keep it off.

But that's not enough. It is not enough that you merely lose weight. What you really have to do is begin to see yourself and think about yourself as a thin person.

You should prepare for this role the same way an actor does when he gets a new part in a play or movie. It will do no good for you to lose 20 or 30 or 40 pounds if you still continue to think and act like a fat person. Because if you do that, one day you will start eating again as a fat person and soon again you will, in fact, actually be fat.

Thin people are more active than fat people. Therefore, I suggest that you become more active. Find yourself a sport that you like and start participating. Or perhaps you might want to take up disco dancing. Buy yourself some new clothes. Make yourself look as good as possible. Flirt a little bit with the opposite sex.

When you go out to eat, don't think of yourself as someone who is deprived. Think of yourself as someone who is lucky enough to be thin and healthy. This will help you resist the things you know you shouldn't eat.

Your friends, or sometimes even your spouse or lover, will exert hidden pressures to get you to gain back the weight you have lost. The reason for this is that they may be uncomfortable with your new attractiveness. Be alert for this. Promise yourself that you are not going to be fat for the rest of your life just because the people around you are more comfortable with the old you.

Be more active. Start going out more. Take up dancing. Get involved in a sport. Buy yourself some new clothes. Take care of your appearance. Start having some fun.

Become a star. Maybe you'll never be in the movies but you can at least be the star of your own life. I know that under the best of circumstances it is hard to diet. My heart is with you. I want you to succeed. Nothing would give me more pleasure than for my publisher to call me up some day and say "Frank, we've got letters from thousands of people who have been helped by your book."

Good luck and God bless you.